Anti-I

Diet

Make these simple, inexpensive changes to your diet and start feeling better within 24 hours!

Written By

Jason Michaels

recorded copy and is only allowed with an expressed written consent from the Publisher. All additional right reserved.

The information in the following pages is broadly considered to be a truthful and accurate account of facts and as such any inattention, use or misuse of the information in question by the reader will render any resulting actions solely under their purview. There are no scenarios in which the publisher or the original author of this work can be in any fashion deemed liable for any hardship or damages that may befall them after undertaking information described herein.

Additionally, the information in the following pages is intended only for informational purposes and should thus be thought of as universal. As befitting its nature, it is presented without assurance regarding its prolonged validity or interim quality. Trademarks that are mentioned are done without written consent and can in no way be considered an endorsement from the trademark holder.

Medical Disclaimer

This book is not intended as a substitute for the medical advice of physicians. The reader should regularly consult a physician in matters relating to his/her health and particularly with respect to any symptoms that may require diagnosis or medical attention.

Please consult your physician before starting any diet or exercise program.

Any recommendations given in this book are not a substitute for medical advice.

Table of Contents

Introduction

Congratulations on downloading *Anti-Inflammatory Diet: Make these simple, inexpensive changes to your diet and start feeling better within 24 hours!* and thank you for doing so.

The following chapters will discuss **how** the anti-inflammatory diet isn't a diet in the traditional meaning of the term, because its intended purpose isn't weight loss, though people do often lose weight when following it. It's also not a diet you follow for a limited time until you reach your goal and then quit. Rather it's a true lifestyle change focused on anti-inflammatory principles with the purpose of providing stable energy, and adequate vitamins, essential fatty acids, minerals, fiber, and defensive anti-inflammatory phytonutrients to reach and maintain better health.

This book is written to help people understand aspects of inflammation and how the typical American diet contributes to it. It looks at the effects of the resulting chronic inflammation on health and how chronic low-grade inflammation can even contribute to weight gain and other health issues. Once equipped with this understanding, you'll learn what you can do about it with a goal to consume less processed and fast foods and more fresh whole foods including plenty of fruits and vegetables. The entire focus of the anti-inflammatory diet is health and healing your body's ailments.

This book also navigates through and beyond misinformation and myths surrounding the diet and lays the groundwork for your new lifestyle. It explains the variety of foods to eat for healing, what foods to avoid, and the best ways to cook meals to get the most benefit. In the end, you'll be equipped with the information you need to get started and to noticeably feel better including a one-week meal plan to get you on track.

There are plenty of books on this subject on the market, thanks again for choosing this one! Every effort was made to ensure it is full of as much useful information as possible, please enjoy!

Thanks,

Jason

Chapter 1: Why the Typical American Diet Is So Bad

Statistics available through the U.S. Department of Health & Human Services (HSS) shine a light on how bad the typical American diet is for us. For starters, "it exceeds the recommended intake levels or limits in four categories: calories from solid fats and added sugars; refined grains; sodium; and saturated fat." All this directly affects your health. In fact, the HSS says that "if Americans reduced the sodium they eat by 1,200 mg per day" going forward "it would save up to $20 billion a year in medical costs." We now get an astonishing 63% of our calories from refined or process foods. And while we eat too much of those foods, on the other end of the spectrum, Americans don't consume the recommended amounts of fruits, vegetables, whole-grains, and healthy oils. In fact, only 12% of our calories coming from plant-based foods. When you look at that statistic even closer, it's even worse because half of that already-low percentage comes from French fries. That means the real number of *healthy* plant-based foods is reduced to 6%, a figure that can only be described as horrifyingly low.

According to the HSS, calories containing no nutrients coming from solid fats and added sugars in the typical American diet "contribute to 40% of the total daily calories for 2 – 18-year-olds and half of these empty calories come from six sources: soda, fruit drinks, dairy desserts, grain desserts, pizza, and whole milk." Forty percent of daily calories! This means almost half of their daily calories contain little or no real nutrients because they are derived from these solid fats and added sugars. And what about the rest of us? Out of a 2775 daily calorie diet, the USDA estimated that in 2010 nearly 1,000 calories a day come from added fats and sweeteners, while only 424 calories came from dairy, fruits, and vegetables.

To better understand what we are talking about, it helps to understand that solid fats are fats that solidify at room temperature. This includes fats like butter, shortening, and fats that cook off of beef, pork, and other meats. Solid fats can be added when foods are processed by manufacturers or when they are prepared for consumption in restaurants or home. In the same way, added sugars include various types of sugars and syrups which are added when foods or beverages are processed or prepared.

In the last 65 years, the amount of sugar we consume has radically gone up, and along with that, the origin of where we get the sugar has also drastically changed. In the 1950s, Americans mostly ate sugar derived from sugarcane and sugar beets, but the year 2000, the USDA reports that each individual in America took in 150 pounds of sugar a year with more than half of that coming from corn in the form of high fructose corn syrup. And no, just because it comes from the plant corn does not make it a sweetener that's good for your health.

Over the last century, our palates have transformed along with the ingredients in our food. Just look at the ingredients list on the foods you buy. Ingredients are listed in the order of prevalence, with ingredients added in the greatest amount listed first, followed in descending order by those in smaller amounts. Sugar in one of its forms is often listed in the first three, because today with the typical American diet everything we eat needs to be really sweet, including foods we don't typically consider sweet such as bread. While sugar is needed to get the yeast to activate and ferment, if you check the label on that multi-grain bread, each slice provides 2.6 grams of sugar from honey and refined sugar.

What's more is, as you read the product label, sugar can be listed by numerous names. These names include anhydrous dextrose, cane juice, corn sweetener, corn syrup, dextrose, fructose, high-fructose corn syrup, corn syrup solids, invert sugar, malt syrup, maltose, lactose, sucrose and white sugar. Unfortunately, food manufacturers aren't required to separate added sugar from naturally occurring sugar but are only required to divulge total over-all sugars per serving.

With the consumption of all these empty calories, today more than 1 in 3 adults suffer from pre-diabetes. This condition happens as the result of higher than "normal" blood sugar levels which aren't at levels bad enough to be identified as type 2 diabetes. Plus, 30 million Americans are inflicted with diabetes but 1 out of 4 aren't even conscious of it.

The bottom line is that Americans aren't taking in enough vital nutrients, fiber, and natural fats needed to attain the best health. This is really sad when you think about how prosperous this great country is and yet we experience higher rates of disease than other developed nations.

What's the cumulative effect of the typical American diet over time? In a nutshell, the standard American diet can lead to chronic inflammation which leads to progressive tissue damage and inflammatory diseases like rheumatoid arthritis and leaky gut. Others ailments include what is known as "unexplained symptoms".

These include things like headaches, brain fog, bleeding gums, allergies, fatigue, mood swings, and skin rashes. In other words, random aches and pains that you can't identify the cause of. In the following chapters, we will take a closer look at chronic low-grade inflammation and what it does to the body. What does this all mean for you? Well simply put, many of your health problems could be caused by nothing more than the food you put into your body on a daily basis. Along with things like causing joint pain, it could well be the reason you're struggling with your weight!

Chapter 2: What Is Chronic Low-Grade Inflammation and Why Does It Make You Fat?

Chronic pain is a growing problem in America. People struggle to get through the day as they battle conditions like arthritis, fibromyalgia, back pain, and more. Many seek relief through strong prescription medication and while this may offer relief, it may also result in unwanted side effects. For those who would rather find another answer, a more natural answer, it's key to understand the connection linking inflammation and pain and the food we put in our mouth. Diets full of things like gluten, trans-fats, pasteurized dairy, corn (including corn sweeteners), and soy are at the source of the pain and inflammation – the same inflammation causing other medical conditions including overweight and obesity.

If you're battling your weight, even though you've cut calories, are exercising regularly and have stopped eating after 8 p.m., have you wondered why you're still carrying all that extra weight around your middle? It just might be that as hard as you are fighting to lose that excess weight, your body is fighting to keep it. Why? Chronic, low-grade inflammation caused by what you are eating.

To understand what one has to do with the other, first, we have to understand chronic inflammation. It is your body's bewildered and detrimental immune response to your environment. Which including poor diet, stress, allergens, and toxic substances. Research shows that what we eat is a significant contributor to chronic inflammation and our gut health. Other factors that contribute to chronic inflammation include a sedentary lifestyle and chronic stress, and living with hidden infections (including things like gum disease).

All these factors trigger this unseen inflammation running deep within our cells and tissues. Think of it like a smoldering fire and when we eat the wrong foods, all we're doing is feeding that fire. And when cytokines that respond to this unseen inflammation fill the bloodstream, it can lead to systemic inflammation, which in turn can lead to cardiovascular diseases. Cholesterol deposits cling to the lining of inflamed blood vessels and grow with a fatty plaque which can lead to blockages and blood clots which in turn can lead to a heart attack.

In this book, we will focus on the dietary link to inflammation, because over time, the continual inflammatory response to our diet is what can lead to weight gain and digestive issues. HHS reports that it is projected that "by 2030, half of all adults (115 million adults) in the United States will be obese." While normal inflammation is a good thing that works to protect and heal your body, chronic or systemic inflammation happens when your immune system gets out of balance and instead of healing, it contributes to disease and weight gain. The sugar we eat contributes to this shift in balance but it isn't the only culprit. Eating the wrong oils and fats including processed seed- and vegetable oils like soybean and corn oil, and hidden food allergens also contribute to the problem.

The influence of food allergens is the culprit directly related to weight gain. We're not talking about life-threatening food allergies some people have to specific foods like peanuts or shellfish, but is a different kind of reaction called a *delayed allergy* (IgG delated hypersensitivity reaction). This kind of deferred response may result in symptoms within a few hours or can be delayed for a few days after eating. This is a much more common allergy and leads millions of people to suffer because it plays a big part in numerous chronic ailments as well as problems with weight. In fact, it's a major contributor to obesity.

So, if you are on the older end of middle age or younger and struggling with your weight even though you think you're doing all the right things, then chronic inflammation could be the cause and an anti-inflammation diet the answer. Eating anti-inflammatory foods eliminates foods containing hidden food allergens and sensitivities, and can help you lose that stubborn weight effectively and permanently as long as you continue to eat the right foods.

Chronic inflammation wears down your immune system over time because it is on-going. As your body continually responds to this inflammation, it eventually leads to chronic diseases and other health issues including:

- Allergies which contribute to sinus and nasal congestion, weight gain, fluid retention, fatigue, joint pains, acne, eczema, brain fog, irritable bowel syndrome (IBS), mood issues, headaches
- Arthritis
- Asthma
- Autoimmune diseases

- Cancer
- Osteoporosis
- Premature aging

Regrettably, most often these chronic health challenges are treated with drugs and/or surgery, which may or may not offer temporary relief from symptoms, but these solutions don't actually address the root of the problem. But if you shop for the right doctor, today you can find an integrative MD who is willing to not only identify health issues but to address them by taking into consideration your lifestyle for ways to eliminate behaviors that lead to chronic inflammation. You can even ask them to run a CRP (C-reactive Protein test) to test your blood for a C-reactive protein which is a blood test marker for inflammation. It forms in the liver and is classified as an "acute phase reactant," which means levels grow higher in as a result of inflammation.

Chapter 3: Anti-Inflammatory Myths

While you can find plenty of information about eating to reduce inflammation, you'll also find plenty of myths and misinformation surrounding the anti-inflammatory diet, too. These myths include warning about foods to avoid as well as foods to eat, along with general all-encompassing statements like everything on the diet tastes terrible, or it's too expensive, so it's important to be informed so you don't sabotage your efforts toward better health before you really get started.

The myths listed in this chapter are deemed so because there's no scientific evidence to support them.

Myth #1: Citrus Fruits Bring About Inflammation

The need to ban citrus fruits because they cause inflammation is one of those unsubstantiated myths circulating on several online forums. The chatter condemns this fruit with little to no scientific evidence to back up claims. In truth, citrus is loaded with vitamin C and proven to reduce the progression of Osteoarthritis. Vitamin C is a beneficial antioxidant and citrus is also known to play an important part in the formation of cartilage.

Myth #2: A Raw Food Diet Alleviates Inflammation

While eating more fruits and vegetables is a good direction to go, eating an all-raw diet isn't necessarily the best solution to fight inflammation. A sudden change in diet like going all raw can actually help promote inflammation instead of relieving it, and the bacteria in your gut may have trouble processing foods so far out of your normal range of choices.

Myth 3: Gin-soaked Raisins Ease Symptoms

This myth is an old wives' tale that finds its origins in the hype surrounding the healing properties of juniper berries which are used to make gin combined with the belief that the sulfur in raisins eases joint pain. And while there may be an inkling of truth in this, it is an unrealistic claim because the amounts typically eaten are so small they make no real impact on your inflammation affecting joints.

Myth #4: Eating a Diet High in Fish Is the Same as Taking AlphaFlex or Fish Oil Supplements

Sorry to say, diet alone can't take the place of AlphaFlex® or other anti-inflammatory supplements. Although the Omega-3's found in fish have anti-inflammatory properties, you would have to eat a large quantity of fish to try to match the anti-inflammatory power of a supplement but you couldn't do it. Plus, fish can also be high in mercury, and excessive consumption could lead to the potential of mercury poisoning.

Myth 5: Eating a low-acid diet helps avoid arthritis flare-ups

The thinking behind this myth says to avoid foods high in acid, like citrus fruits and tomatoes to minimize pain and flare-ups. The problem with this is that as you eat and drink gets balanced once it enters your stomach. The digestive system adjusts foods whether acidic and alkaline and neutralizes and supposed benefit or detriment based on those qualifiers. Plus, citrus fruits are high in vitamin C which works as an anti-inflammatory.

Myth 6: Making Healthier Choices Is Cost Prohibitive

And one more myth related to following the anti-inflammatory diet is that healthier choices are cost prohibitive. It is true that processed foods filled with added sugars and higher fat content do cost less monetarily than nutrient-dense whole fruits, vegetables, lean meats. In fact, fresh vegetable and fruit prices rose almost 120% from 1985 – 2000. With those kinds of statistics, it does seem like making healthier choices is just too expensive for some of us. But that's really not the case.

Findings in a recent meta-analysis by researchers at Brown University and the Harvard School of Public Health shine a light on just how much more expensive it really is to buy healthier food options. They crunched numbers from 27 previous studies and what did they find? The cost for an adult to eat healthy comes to $1.48 a day more than eating a poor-quality diet. That calculates out to $550 more per person a year. Isn't that worth it for better health?

There are a few ways that can help you save more when eating a healthy anti-inflammatory diet. One of the big ones is to eat out less and to cook for yourself more. For instance, people spend an average of $11 per meal eating lunch out, but only $6.30 on average when they prepare their own lunch, plus when you make your own food you have the added benefit of knowing exactly what is in it. Also, as you increase the amount of fruits and vegetables in your diet, you'll find if you buy them in season you'll get the best value.

One last myth worth mentioning, even though it doesn't have anything to do with food and nutrition, is that *all anti-inflammatory medications have minimal side effects*. Sadly, the opposite is true. Even anti-inflammatory over-the-counter drugs like ibuprofen, naproxen, Celebrex and other non-steroidal drugs can result in a number of side effects, plus these drugs really need to be taken in prescription doses to curb inflammation.

These possible side effects include ulcers that may possibly become life-threatening, abdominal pain, diarrhea, dry mouth, kidney failure, swelling, and dizziness. On the flip side, fish oil is a natural supplement that fights inflammation without any known adverse side effects.

When searching for a fish oil, you should choose one that has the optimal EPA/DHA ratio. Ideally you want a supplement with 180mg EPA and 120mg DHA per serving.

Chapter 4: Top 7 Foods to Avoid

When eating to reduce inflammation, it is best to avoid most packaged foods because they contain inflammation-triggering preservatives, colorings, and artificial flavorings to increase their shelf life. If it is packaged in a box or bag, chances are that it's not good for your health. Eating too many inflammatory foods can lead to chronic low-grade inflammation which in turn can cause serious health issues including cancer, heart disease, diabetes, and allergies. With that said, this chapter looks at seven specific inflammatory foods to avoid.

1. Gluten and Wheat

As we've already discussed, inflammation is the natural response of your immune system. When we get a splinter, inflammation makes the surrounding area red and tender. With this picture in mind, let's look at why you should avoid gluten.

Proteins found in wheat are gut irritants, and the term "gluten" is a general name for these proteins. Now, picture tiny splinters raking into the lining of your gut and resulting in inflammation. When it comes to gluten, the most well-known gluten-related inflammation is celiac disease or non-celiac gluten sensitivity, but wheat can also be a problem for people who aren't specifically sensitive to gluten because of amylase trypsin inhibitors (ATIs) found in wheat. These ATIs can bring about an inflammatory immune response in the GI tract which contributes to another problem called intestinal permeability, or leaky gut, which we will cover more in chapter 8. This condition lets undigested food particles, bacteria, and toxic waste products "leak" through the intestines into your bloodstream.

2. Refined Carbohydrates

Carbohydrates are commonly referred to as "good" and "bad." Complex carbs are *good* because they are filled with beneficial fiber. When it comes to inflammation, refined carbohydrates fall into the bad category because in the refining process most of their fiber is removed. With the fiber removed, refined carbs raise blood sugar levels and raise the occurrence of inflammatory changes. This influence can lead to disease. For instance, when looking at our modern diet, research has shown refined carbs can encourage the development of inflammatory bacteria in the gut which can raise the probability of obesity and IBS.

3. Milk Lactose

Milk lactose is a sugar found in milk which causes digestive issues for many people because their bodies don't produce the lactase enzyme required to digest it. Other people who do produce this enzyme may still react poorly to drinking milk because of the proteins casein and whey. Casein actually has a molecular structure very similar to gluten, and half the people who can't tolerate gluten don't tolerate casein well either. As a result, dairy is one of the most inflammatory foods in today's diet, second only to gluten. Adverse digestive symptoms resulting from this inflammation may manifest in bloating, constipation, diarrhea, and gas. Other non-digestive symptoms include acne and a compelling demonstration of autistic behaviors. So lactose is only half the issue when it comes to milk and milk products, the others are the casein and whey proteins.

A study also showed that women in China have a far lower rate of breast cancer than women in the West. The only noticeable difference between the two diets is lower milk intake. A Harvard professor has also discovered links between ovarian cancer and dairy consumption.

4. Sugar

It's no secret that eating too many added sugars and refined carbohydrates can lead to overweight and obesity, but the consequences of eating excesses are also linked to increased gut permeability, raised inflammatory markers, and high LDL cholesterol. The thing all these factors have in common is that they can trigger low-grade chronic inflammation. Excess body fat, especially belly fat, results in continuous, chronic levels of inflammation which can modify how insulin works. Insulin, as a regulatory hormone, plays a big part in carrying the glucose in your bloodstream into your cells for energy, but when blood glucose levels are chronically high, the production and regulation of insulin is changed resulting in insulin resistance. The resulting overabundance of blood glucose can lead to an accumulation of advanced glycation end products (AGEs). When too many AGEs bind with our cells and integral proteins, it can lead to oxidative stress and inflammation. It can change their structure, inhibit their regular function and eventually result in a buildup of arterial plaque and decreased kidney function, among other things.

5. Meat

Grain fed beef has been touted as tasting better, but cows are naturally grazers that eat grass. When fed grain they grow fat quickly before they are sold by the pound for profit. Cattle, pigs, and chickens are not naturally grain eaters. But in life on the feed-lot not only are they fed things like corn and soy, they are also given antibiotics to make sure they don't get sick. This translates to meats on our dinner table that are not only higher in inflammatory saturated fats but also contain higher levels of inflammatory omega-6s from their unnatural diet. To compound the problem, when we grill our meat at high temperatures, it results in inflammatory carcinogens! So if you plan to eat meat, choose grass-fed varieties.

.

6. Saturated Fats

When you think saturated fats, many people think of red meat, but aside from fatty cuts of beef, saturated fat is also found in pork and lamb, the skin of chicken, as well as processed meats. It's also found in dairy products like butter, cream (including whipped cream), cheese, and regular-fat milk. Studies have linked the consumption of saturated fats with causing the kind of body fat that stores energy rather than burns it. As these fat cells grow bigger they release pro-inflammatory drivers that promote systemic inflammation.

7. Alcohol

Drinking alcohol puts a burden on the liver, and when consumed in excess, it weakens liver function. This disrupts other multi-organ interactions resulting in inflammation. If you choose to drink alcohol, do so in moderation, but it is best eliminated if you're fighting inflammation.

Chapter 5: Most Beneficial Foods and Best Anti-inflammatory Supplements

Many conditions can be traced back to inflammation. Joint pain, autoimmune disorders, irritable bowel syndrome (IBS), mood imbalances, acne, and eczema are just a few conditions that can be linked back to inflammation. Once the origin of inflammation is identified, an anti-inflammatory diet can help ease symptoms and certain foods and supplements can help lessen the inflammation in your body. In this chapter, we'll list some of the best minerals and beneficial antioxidants found in foods and supplements to add to your arsenal to fight inflammation. This list is arranged in alphabetical order to make it easier to use as a reference tool.

Blueberries

Blueberries make the list as an antioxidant superfood. This dark, delicious fruit may be small, but it's crammed with antioxidants and phytoflavinoids. These tiny berries are high in potassium and vitamin C and work as an anti-inflammatory to aid in lowering the risk of heart disease and cancer. They also assist with preventing mental decline. Strawberries, raspberries, and blackberries also contain anthocyanins which provide anti-inflammatory effects.

Avocado

Avocados are packed with potassium, magnesium, and fiber. This savory fruit is another superfood rich in antioxidants and anti-inflammatory properties. They provide a great source of healthy unsaturated fat and are packed with potassium, magnesium, and fiber.

Coenzyme Q10

Coenzyme Q10, also known as CoQ10, is another antioxidant that shown to offer anti-inflammatory properties. It is found naturally in avocados, olive oil, parsley, peanuts, beef liver, salmon, sardines, mackerel, spinach, and walnuts.

Ginger

Ginger is comparative to in that contains powerful anti-inflammatory compounds known as gingerols. Ginger root is found in the produce section at your grocery store and is available as a potent antioxidant supplement that helps prevent the oxidation of a damaging free radical called peroxynitrite. Ginger adds flavor to your favorite stir-fry, can be made into ginger tea, or can be taken as a supplement.

Glutathione

Glutathione is another antioxidant that fights free-radicals with anti-inflammatory properties. This is available as a supplement and is also available naturally in plant foods including apples, asparagus, avocados, garlic, grapefruit, spinach, tomatoes, and milk thistle.

Magnesium

Magnesium is a mineral supplement that can help reduce inflammation for those with low magnesium which is linked to stress. Statistics suggest an estimated 70% of Americans are deficient in this mineral which is surprising since it is readily available in a number of foods including dark leafy greens, almonds, avocado, and many legumes.

Salmon

Salmon is rich in anti-inflammatory omega-3s. It is better to eat wild caught than farmed. It is best to try to include oily fish in your diet two times a week, and if you're not a fan of fish, then try a high-quality fish oil supplement.

Turmeric/Curcumin

Turmeric is the yellow spice that gives curry its color, and curcumin is the active ingredient in turmeric and can be purchased as a supplement. The two words are often used interchangeably, but curcumin is the key ingredient which offers powerful anti-inflammatory effects. It's a strong antioxidant and as a powdered spice, turmeric can be added to soups and curries, and curcumin can be taken in supplement form.

Vitamin B

People with low levels of vitamin B6 have a tendency to have high levels of C-reactive protein which, as was mentioned in chapter 2, is a measure of inflammation in the body. B vitamins, including B6, can be found in vegetables like broccoli, bell peppers, cauliflower, kale, and mushrooms. It is also available in meats including chicken, cod, turkey, and tuna.

Folate (B-9 in natural form) and folic acid (a synthetic form of B-9) is another B vitamin linked to the reduction of inflammation. A brief Italian study submits that even daily, short-term low dosages of folic acid supplements can lessen inflammation in overweight people. Folate is found in foods like asparagus, black-eyed peas, dark leafy greens, and lima beans.

Vitamin D

Estimates suggest two-thirds of the people living in the U.S. are deficient in vitamin D. It's another vitamin that helps reduce inflammation, and getting insufficient amounts is linked to a range of inflammatory conditions. This vitamin is unique in that we get it naturally when we spend time in the sunshine with the important spectrum is ultraviolet B (UVB). It is also available as a supplement and is available in foods like egg yolks, fish and organ meats, as well as foods that are supplemented with it. When choosing a Vitamin D supplement, look for

Vitamin D3, which is the most bioavailable form of the vitamin. The ideal amount for supplementation is 5000IU per day, and many of this pills cost less than $7 for a 3 month supply.

Vitamin E

Another potent antioxidant, this vitamin can aid in lessening inflammation. It is available as a quality supplement or can be found naturally in nuts and seeds, and vegetables like avocado and spinach.

Vitamin K

There are two kinds of vitamin K: K1 and K2. K1 is found in leafy greens, cabbage, and cauliflower. K2 is available in eggs and liver. This vitamin helps reduce inflammatory markers and may help to fight osteoporosis and heart disease.

Chapter 6: How to Extract the Most Nutrients from Your Food When Cooking

For decades, raw foodists have warned that cooking not only kills vitamins and minerals in food but also denatures the enzymes that help us digest the foods we eat. We've heard this for so long, many of us had embraced it as fact, but the truth is raw vegetables aren't always healthier, and in some cases, cooking is actually important if we want to get the most nutritional benefit from the foods we eat. Cooking can help us digest food without spending volumes of energy and makes foods like cellulose fiber and raw meat softer for and easier for our digestive systems to handle.

It turns out that vegetables like asparagus, cabbage, carrots, peppers, mushrooms, spinach, and numerous others, actually supply our bodies with more antioxidants like carotenoids and ferulic acid when boiled or steamed as opposed to raw. A January 2008 report in the Journal of

Agriculture and Food Chemistry reported that when cooking vegetables "boiling and steaming preserved antioxidants better than frying." This was mainly the case with carotenoid present in broccoli, carrots, and zucchini. And before you shrug it off and say, "Any cooking method is better than frying," it's important to note that researchers actually examined the effect of several cooking methods on compounds such as carotenoids, polyphenols, and ascorbic acid and determined boiling to be the best way to extract these nutrients for consumption.

In the same year, a study published in The British Journal of Nutrition backed up this cooking benefit claim. This study consisted of a group of 198 participants and found those who adhered to an inflexible raw food diet showed normal quantities of vitamin A and comparatively elevated levels of beta-carotene. However, they had low levels of the antioxidant lycopene, a carotenoid with anti-inflammatory properties. Remember, these are findings for eating raw. In contrast, another study published in the Journal of Agriculture and Food Chemistry found that cooking essentially raises the quantity of lycopene in tomatoes. "The level of one type of lycopene, cis-lycopene, rose 35% after being cooked for 30 minutes at 190.4 degrees Fahrenheit." The conclusions drawn suggest that heat causes the thick cell walls of the plant to break down which aids in the body's absorption of nutrients which were bound to those cell walls. So now that we know some nutrition is enhanced by cooking but not everything is best cooked, it leaves us with the question: "What should I cook and what should I eat raw on the anti-inflammatory diet?" The fact is that each food is a little different. The raw foodist mentality holds that many foods high in antioxidants are sensitive to cooking because phytonutrients don't hold up well to high temperatures and when it reaches the "heat labile point" it results in a change that causes foods to lose enzymes beneficial to us. But this is only half the story. The truth is that whether you should eat a vegetable cooked or raw for the most nutritional benefit depends on the vegetable and the way you cook it.

Jason Michaels

The hidden dangers of microwaving

Before we go any further, let's be clear – deep frying offers no benefit, and microwaving your food can actually bring about an inflammatory response. This is because microwaving brings about a change in the chemical structure of your food. In fact, it so completely alters the protein structure of food that the body doesn't even recognize it as a food, but instead looks at as a foreign toxin which warrants an inflammatory response.

Microwaving food is also harmful to nutritive benefit and leads to a loss of up to 90% of the nutritional value. It converts tasty, organic vegetables into nutritionally "dead" food that can bring about disease because microwaving changes plant alkaloids into carcinogens. Take garlic for example. It's a powerful healing food when eaten raw and is of great benefit to digestive health, cellular immunity, heart health and more, but when microwaved for just 60 seconds the active component, allinase, become inactive. So the very component known to help protect against cancer is no longer any benefit at all.

The same kinds of changes occur when microwaving grains and milk, too. In these cases, the amino acids are converted into carcinogenic substances. When it comes to prepared meats microwaving again results in the development of cancer-causing agents. And if you use the microwave to thaw frozen fruits, it causes the sugar molecule to break down into carcinogenic substances.

An additional concern deals with carcinogenic toxins which can leach out of plastic containers, lids, or wraps used when microwaving. One of the nastiest contaminants is BPA which can cause chaos with our natural hormone levels. Often, BPAs can overstimulate the manufacture of oestrogen which can lead to oestrogenic cancers. So the next time you think about popping your food into the microwave, remember that microwaving results in molecular damage which not only kills nutritional benefits, but in its wake, leaves carcinogenic substances. So while it can seem convenient to rapidly heat your food, microwaving is not worth the nutritional loss or risk to your health.

Cooking with light heat or steam is the best as it breaks down food making it release easier-to-absorb nutrients. In some cases, as we've seen, it can even increase the nutrient content available. Another benefit related to cooking is that it can also transform chemicals from being potentially harmful to harmless. But, it depends on the vegetable and the method of cooking.

With all this in mind, the following list of vegetables is the ones better eaten cooked.

Asparagus:

The best way to cook asparagus is to steam or blanch it or bake it in a casserole. The process breaks down the fibrous spears making them easier to digest and allowing easier absorption of nutrients including vitamins A, B, C, E, and K.

Broccoli:

Finding the best way to cook broccoli is a little trickier. Those who have hypothyroidism, shouldn't eat your broccoli raw because it contains a thyroid-disrupting element. Steaming lets you preserve the nutrients while leaching out some of this element. Also, to retain a healthy amount of beneficial elements of broccoli, it helps to chop it before steaming. Avoid microwaving or boiling.

Carrots:

Carrots are best cooked by roasting or steaming. As the study mentioned earlier revealed, cooking your carrots can significantly raise the bioavailability of beta-carotene which is converted to vitamin A in our bodies. When you eat carrots raw, it's not absorbed as well.

Red Peppers:

When preparing red peppers roasting is the most advantageous. These vegetables are a remarkable source of carotenoids. And, like carrots, cooking can enhance the bioavailability of these carotenoids. However, don't overcook because it can destroy heat-sensitive antioxidants.

Spinach:

Dark green spinach leaves make a popular salad choice, but it turns out this is another vegetable that is better eaten cooked. Nutritionally, it's best to steam it. Because it wilts when steamed, one cup steamed holds more actual spinach as well as nutrients than one cup raw. But there's another cooking benefit related to the oxalic acid found in spinach. Oxalic acid hampers the absorption of certain minerals including calcium and iron and can even develop kidney stones. But cooking spinach reduces oxalic acid by 5—53%, and if you boil it, the percentage lost rises to 30—37%. However, steaming is better unless you are prone to kidney stones because boiling leaches folate from spinach leaves. Spinach is also advisable if you have a history of heart disease in the family.

Tomatoes:

Tomatoes are a rich source of lycopene which offers both anti-inflammatory and antioxidant properties and it, too, becomes more bioavailable after cooking. Just cook them with a little olive oil, or reduce tomatoes down to a sauce, tomato puree, or ketchup to notably increase the absorption of lycopene.

Chapter 7: Foods You Wouldn't Have Thought Were Good for You

It isn't uncommon when starting a diet to think, you'll have to give up everything you like, but with the anti-inflammatory diet, you may be pleasantly surprised to find there are delicious anti-inflammatory food and drinks options on the menu that you wouldn't have thought good for you.

Dark Chocolate

Let's start with chocolate. It not only makes for a special treat, it is actually good for you! When choosing chocolate with anti-inflammatory benefits look for chocolate that contains at least 70% cocoa (at the minimum). Along with being loaded with antioxidants that reduce inflammation, it may also lead to healthier aging because the flavonoids found in dark chocolate modify the production of a pro-inflammatory cytokine. Research suggests eating dark chocolate regularly or even occasionally can bring about beneficial results on blood pressure, oxidative stress, vascular damage, and insulin resistance.

Coffee

More than half of people in the United States drink coffee every day, but should we? Turns out coffee is actually the chief source of antioxidants in American diets. So it's okay to look forward to that cup of coffee in the morning for more than one reason whether it's decaf or regular because it contains polyphenols and other anti-inflammatory compounds. Numerous studies back this up, but one published in 2015 discovered that "over 30 years, nonsmokers who drank 3 to 5 cups of coffee a day were 15 percent less likely to die of any cause compared to people who didn't drink coffee." The coffee drinkers showed lower rates of death from heart disease, stroke, and neural conditions.

However, there is a downside to drinking coffee for some people as it causes some to experience insomnia, anxiety, irregular heartbeat and other negative side effects like irritation of the digestive system. If you experience any downside to drinking coffee, then it is best to avoid it. Try tea instead.

Tea

Green tea is another good-for-you beverage option. Of the many green teas available, Matcha tea is the most nutrient-rich. It offers up to 17 times more antioxidants than found in wild blueberries, and seven times more than what is in dark chocolate. What may surprise you, though, is that green, white or black tea all enjoy potent anti-inflammatory benefits. So if you're not a fan of green tea, you can drink the tea of your choice and still get the potent anti-inflammatory benefits of catechin polyphenols.

Garlic and Onions

Garlic and onions bring plenty of flavor to the anti-inflammatory food palate. Garlic has a long history as a staple folk treatment for colds and other illness. It provides sulfur compounds that encourage the immune system to battle disease. Garlic has been shown to work in the same way as over the counter nonsteroidal anti-inflammatory pain drugs like ibuprofen, by reducing pathways that lead to inflammation.

Onions provide comparable anti-inflammatory compounds, one of which is the phytonutrient quercetin, which breaks down to create free radical-fighting sulfenic acid. Crushing and chopping garlic and onion releases the enzyme alliinase, which helps form a nutrient called allicin. When consumed, allicin helps form other compounds that may protect us against disease.

Fermented Foods

If you're new to fermented foods they open a whole new experience in taste. Kombucha is a fermented lightly sweetened effervescent drink that's fermented. It's made with black or green tea and boasts a host of health benefits. You can buy kombucha in the cooler section of many stores, or if you're a DIY person, you can buy a kit or active Kombucha Scoby and you're your own. Along with kombucha, fermented dishes or products to try include kefir, miso, and sauerkraut. These cultured foods provide healthy bacteria which will optimize your gut health and support a healthy immune system, which in turn helps to reduce inflammation in the body.

In some ways, learning to follow an anti-inflammatory diet is a journey as you unlearn past behaviors and reinvent your tastes as to what is really good. Keep nuts like nuts like almonds and walnuts on hand for a go-to snack along with a selection of fruits like strawberries, blueberries, cherries, pineapple, and oranges.

Strawberries in particular are great if you're searching for a flat stomach. These delicious berries are packed with polyphenols which a study by the Texas Women's University found decreased the formation of fat cells in the stomach by up to 73%.

Yes, making changes to avoid inflammation does take some work and a change in thinking, and in some cases a change in the preferences of your taste buds, but when you realize you can enjoy foods you really like that actually heal your body and improve your health and even your mood and can save you money on drugs, you'll embrace the change.

Chapter 8: Healing Foods for Leaky Gut, Arthritis, and Other Associated Disease

We've talked about how the anti-inflammatory diet is a healing diet and, in this chapter, we will take a closer look at what that really means for people with leaky gut and arthritis. For many of us, looking at inflammation as a root cause is a new concept, because traditionally modern medicine treats it as a symptom. For instance, we know arthritis is inflammation of the joints. The common answer is to take medication to reduce inflammation, but that's only treating the symptom and isn't really addressing the real problem – what's causing the inflammation. When health professionals discuss an anti-inflammatory diet, this type of low-grade, chronic inflammation is what they normally expect to help.

Before we take a closer look at arthritis and what anti-inflammatory foods to eat to specifically to help combat that condition, we will discuss another condition that can leave you feeling depressed, fatigued, anxious, struggling with weight problems or digestive symptoms. We're talking about leaky gut syndrome which is also identified as increased intestinal permeability. It's a dangerous health condition in which your digestive tract gets damaged and permits bad bacteria, proteins like gluten, and undigested bits of food to pass into your bloodstream. Some of the early symptoms of leaky gut can include skin conditions like acne and eczema, food allergies, and digestive issues including bloating, gas and irritable bowel syndrome (IBS). Over time leaky gut causes systemic inflammation and an immune reaction. It's been associated with chronic diseases and conditions including asthma, autism, chronic fatigue syndrome, depression, diabetes, heart failure, IBS, infertility, kidney disease, lupus, multiple sclerosis, narcolepsy, psoriasis, rheumatoid arthritis, and more.

Most people don't begin to understand the role our intestines play in our overall health. The small intestine absorbs the majority of the vitamins and minerals from the foods we eat. For this absorption to take place, the small intestine is equipped with tiny pores that allow nutrients to be transferred into the bloodstream. The bloodstream works as a conduit that carries and deposits these nutrients around the body. Because the intestine has these tiny pores, the wall of the intestine is referred to as semi-permeable because it permits specific things like nutrients and other beneficial molecules to enter the bloodstream while blocking things like toxins and undigested food particles.

An unhealthy small intestine suffering from leak gut no longer works properly because the pores widen and allow harmful things to pass into your bloodstream and to be transported throughout the body. Often the body starts to recognize certain foods as toxic which results in an immune reaction every time you eat that food. If the problem goes on unchecked, leaky gut can advance to an autoimmune disease. To repair this increased intestinal permeability specific diet changes must be made.

Foods to Eat to Support Healing Leaky Gut

Foods that help leaky gut are easy to digest and can aid in healing the lining of the intestines:

Bone broth: Delivers important amino acids and minerals that can aid in healing heal leaky gut and improve mineral deficits. Best if made from scratch.

Probiotic-rich foods: Raw cultured dairy products like yogurt, kefir, and amasai can help heal the gut by wiping out bad bacteria.

Healthy fats: Consume healthy fats found in foods like avocados, egg yolks, coconut oil, salmon, and ghee in moderation. These fats promote healing and are easy on the gut.

Fermented vegetables: Foods like sauerkraut, kimchi, coconut kefir, or kvass contain probiotics vital in mending leaky gut by balancing the pH in the stomach and small intestines.

Steamed vegetables: Steamed non-starchy vegetables are easy to digest and a crucial part of the leaky gut diet.

Fruit: Fruit should be eaten in moderation; 1-2 servings each day. Best to eat it in the morning.

Foods to Eat to Support Arthritis

When the body is inflamed, C-reactive protein levels (CRP) rise, so if present it's a clear indicator of inflammation. Doctors can order a test checking for CRPs. According to studies published in *Molecular Nutrition & Food Research* and in the *Journal of Nutrition*, whole grains such as brown rice, bulgur, quinoa, and others have been linked with reduced CRP levels. Another study in the Journal of Nutrition discovered that people who ate smaller amounts of whole grains essentially experienced higher inflammation markers. According to the Arthritis Foundation, the fiber available in whole grains like oats can help resolve inflammatory processes by helping to achieve weight loss and by nourishing valuable gut bacteria linked with lower levels of inflammation and help soothe IBS. What we eat can make a difference in the inflammation associated with arthritis.

Types of Anti-inflammatory Foods to Eat to Help Arthritis

Foods Rich in Omega-3: Wild-caught fish, including salmon, is your best choice for omega-3 fats. Other foods to include in your diet include chia seeds, flax seeds, grass-fed beef, and walnuts.

Foods Rich in Sulfur: Sulfur boosts antioxidants and can help repair joints. Foods rich in sulfur include broccoli, brussels sprouts, cabbage, cauliflower, chives, collard greens, garlic, onions, garlic, grass-fed beef, leeks, organic eggs, radishes, raw dairy, watercress and wild-caught fish.

Bone Broth: Bone broth also makes the list for your arthritis diet because of its remarkable healing properties. According to nutrition researchers from the Weston A. Price Foundation, bone broth contains chondroitin sulfates and glucosamine which are the very compounds available in costly supplements designed to decrease joint pain and inflammation.

Fruits and Vegetables: Like every anti-inflammatory diet, fruits and vegetables are an important component. They provide digestive enzymes as well as anti-inflammatory compounds. When it comes to arthritis two of the best to be sure to include in your diet are papaya, which contains papain, and pineapple, which contains bromelain which research has shown may aid in decreasing disease-causing inflammation with ailments like rheumatoid arthritis.

Chapter 9: Anti-Inflammatory Herbs

Chronic inflammation is long-term. It results from the failure to eliminate whatever is causing the original acute inflammation and can last for months or even years. When people have inflammation, it often results in pain because of biochemical progressions that occur during inflammation leading to swelling that presses against sensitive nerve endings. This influences how nerves behave and can enhance pain. As a result, the kind of pain varies from one person to another and might come in the form of stiffness, discomfort, and even agony, but the thing sufferers have in common is that the pain is constant. It might be described as steady throbbing, stabbing, or pinching. Symptoms of chronic inflammation present in a number of ways including abdominal pain, chest pain, fatigue, fever, joint pain, mouth sores, muscle weakness and sometimes pain, and rashes.

Because of the side effects associated with traditional painkillers, many are turning to more natural herbal methods for healing and pain management. We've mentioned a handful of herbs and herbal supplements in earlier chapters, but here we dedicate the entire chapter to anti-inflammatory herbs. However, before you include herbal supplements in your health regime, it is best to talk with your doctor or pharmacist regarding any possible interactions with prescription or over-the-counter medications you may be taking.

Cayenne pepper:

The health benefits of cayenne and other hot chili peppers have been recognized since ancient times. Natural compounds called capsaicinoids are found in cayenne and all chili peppers. It's what gives them their spice and anti-inflammatory properties.

Black pepper:

The sharp taste of black pepper makes it one of the most popular spices in the world, but the piperine compound that gives black pepper that taste so many love is also a compound that prevents inflammation and makes it effective in reducing symptoms of arthritis.

Cinnamon:

Cinnamon is a common but popular spice often used to add flavor baked treats, but studies have shown it offers so much more than good flavor. This spice is rich in antioxidants, helps the body fight infection, and has anti-inflammatory properties which can ease swelling and repair tissue damage. Sprinkle it in your coffee or tea for a touch of flavor as just one way to enjoy its healing benefits.

Cloves:

Cloves are a pungent spice known for its anti-inflammatory properties. Researchers at the University of Florida conducted a study that had participants consume cloves daily and found that in just seven days it significantly lowered one specific pro-inflammatory cytokine. Because of its strong flavor, cloves pair well with nutmeg and cinnamon to add a tasty kick to stews and means. It's also a popular addition to Indian cuisine.

Devil's Claw:

This herb originally comes from South Africa and has been a remedy for African and European traditional and folk doctors used for centuries to treat digestive problems, relieve pain, reduce fever, and to treat some pregnancy symptoms. It also goes by the names wood spider or the grapple plant and it makes a popular choice for people suffering from arthritis and other forms of joint or back pain when combined with bromelain. In supplement form, devil's claw is derived from the dried roots of the plant. Research has shown it may have anti-inflammatory properties.

Ginger:

We talked about ginger as a supplement in chapter 5, but garlic in its natural form has been used for hundreds of years to treat things like constipation, sinus congestion, indigestion, colic and other digestive problems, as well as rheumatoid arthritis pain. When taken orally, garlic is said to be beneficial for helping with pain and arthritis. Cloves can be eaten raw or cooked, or it can be purchased as a supplement in powdered form in capsules or tablets. It's also available in liquid extracts and oils.

Rosemary:

Rosemary leaves are often used in cooking, but this herb is much more than an aromatic plant. It provides a whole range of possible health benefits. It's plentiful in antioxidants and anti-inflammatory compounds believed to aid in boosting the immune system.

Sage:

The medicinal use of sage goes way back. In the past, it's been used for ailments ranging from mental disorders to intestinal and digestive discomfort. In more recent years, studies show the health benefits of sage have grown since then. Not it appears to contain a range of anti-inflammatory and antioxidant compounds and research has reinforced some of its medical applications. Along with use in cooking, it is commonly used to make sage tea as a way to enjoy its many benefits.

Spirulina:

Spirulina is a blue-green algae and considered a superfood. It's a rich source of vitamin B12, full of antioxidants, and is approximately 62% amino acids. Research has established that Spirulina prevents the production and release of histamine, which is a chemical that kindles an inflammatory response in the body. Additional research confirms that Spirulina may lessen arthritis. However, Spirulina is not recommended for those who suffer from digestive issues because it is very difficult to digest.

Chapter 10: Start Feeling Better Instantly

Since we've covered how inflammation works, the health problems surrounding chronic inflammation, and the foods to eat to combat those problems, in this chapter we will discuss the benefits associated with eating a more plant-based diet along with other lifestyle aspects needed to help fight your way back to good health.

Growing evidence shows diet and lifestyle can either generate a pro-inflammatory environment or an anti-inflammatory environment. So, if you are suffering from chronic inflammation you can quickly start feeling better than you do at this moment by making lifestyle changes right now. The first step in is to start choosing the right foods, but it's more than that. Buying the right foods won't make a difference if you don't prepare them correctly. For that reason, it's just as important to learn how to prepare those foods using anti-inflammatory cooking methods (see chapter 6). If you don't, you can undo the very healthy benefits you're hoping to enjoy.

Remember, your daily food selections are the source of your chronic inflammation. To jumpstart your anti-inflammatory diet, embrace a more plant-based diet because when it comes to fighting chronic inflammation, one of the biggest benefits of consuming a plant-based diet is its ability to lower chronic inflammation levels. In fact, it is suggested that inflammation might just be the biggest reason why plant-based diets have been shown to promote health while our typical American diet promotes disease. To be clear, "plant-based" doesn't necessarily me no meat, because it can allow for limited quantities of fish and lean meat. What it does mean is a diet heavy in nutrient-dense vegetables and fruits that can aid in warding off inflammation and disease. In 2014 study on diet and inflammatory bowel disease, 33% of the participants in the study opted not to go with the proposed anti-inflammatory diet. The participants who did decide to follow the anti-inflammatory diet experienced enough relief that they could discontinue at least one of their medications.

Nutrient dense foods offer high levels of vitamins, minerals, and/or protein per serving. If you want to jumpstart your anti-inflammatory diet to start feeling better faster, along with buying and preparing nutrient-dense foods and preparing them properly, it's also important to stay hydrated, but to keep costs down your should drink tap water instead of bottled - unless you cannot drink the tap water in your area. Avoid chlorinated, waters because you're working to eliminate substances you don't need in your body. Staying hydrated helps to suppress cellular inflammation and will decrease inflammation in the body.

Along with taking care of what you put into your body, it's also important that you get regular adequate exercise. Doing so can actually boost your immune system. Not being active enough is actually hard on your body, but be careful to not overdo it. Plan 20-30 minutes of light to moderate exercise most day. With physical activity comes free radical damage and the breaking down of body tissue. This results in some low-level inflammation in the body as it heals during the recovery time between active times. So the goal is to find the middle ground. To be active, but not overactive. To move enough, but to rest enough. If you don't do this, it can result in inflammation to build up.

As the repairing and restoring process works within the body while you sleep, it's hard at work. For this reason, getting enough rest is important with doctors recommending 7 to 8 hours of sleep per night. If you're lacking in sleep, you're taking advantage of your immune system. As a result, it needs to work harder to try to keep you well. Lack of sleep leads to stress. Constant stress produces more cortisol and you guessed it, inflammation. So as you work to eat right, you need to put in the effort to also be active enough and to get your rest. It really is a lifestyle.

Chapter 11: Anti-inflammatory Meal Plan for 1 Week

As you reach toward better health going forward, your new goal is to consume a variety of nutrient-dense whole foods that can reduce inflammation. Making this move doesn't have to be hard, and it doesn't have to be expensive. You have plenty of foods to choose from and when you buy fruits and vegetable in season you will often find they cost less than a dollar per serving. The following list offers examples of anti-inflammatory foods that cost under a dollar per serving using in-season produce prices.

- Apples: $0.75 each
- Broccoli: $0.50 per 1/2 cup, $1.99 per bunch
- Cage-free Eggs: $0.25 per egg based on $2.99 a dozen
- Canned salmon: $0.80 for 4 oz. serving, based on $2.50 for 14.75 oz. can

- Cantaloupe: $0.50 for 1/2 cup, $3 per small melon and in season you can find them for much less
- Carrots: $0.50 each at $2 per pound
- Chicken breast: $0.75 for a 4-ounce serving, $2.99 per pound
- Garlic: $0.30 per bulb
- Grapes: $0.75 per cup, $1.50 per pound
- Kiwi: $0.40 each
- Mandarin oranges: $0.23 per piece, $3.99 for 5 pounds
- Onions: $0.18 each, $0.59 per pound
- Whole grain oats: $0.13 per serving, $3.98 for 30 oz. container. You can find oats for even less if you buy in bulk.

When you stop and really consider how many servings you get for your money when buying healthy foods, cost shouldn't really be a deterrent.

Sample Meal Plan for One Week

Day 1

Breakfast: Scrambled eggs served with chopped cabbage and onions seasoned with cumin seeds and turmeric. Steam until cabbage is softened but lightly crisp.

Lunch: Grilled salmon served on a bed of spring greens with olive oil and vinegar.

Dinner: Chicken breast seasoned with fresh herbs, and zesty lemon, steamed broccoli, and a serving of steamed brown rice.

Snack: 1 cup frozen grapes

Day 2

Breakfast: Oats (high in fiber, low in fat, oats contain *avenanthramides* which play a role in reducing inflammation). Add fruit like sliced banana or fresh dark-colored berries and a handful of walnuts.

Lunch: Spiced lentil soup seasoned with cinnamon, cayenne pepper, cumin, turmeric, and cayenne pepper

Dinner: Salmon patty (made using canned salmon, eggs, garlic, shallot, ginger, coconut flour, walnuts, cumin, turmeric, salt, and pepper), garden salad, topped with your favorite anti-inflammatory dressing.

Snack: Turmeric Chai Chia Pudding (from The Blenderist)

Day 3

Breakfast: Poached eggs served on fat-free refried beans topped with fresh salsa with sliced avocado on the side.

Lunch: Blueberry Banana smoothie made with coconut water and frozen banana

Dinner: Chicken curry made with sweet potato, broccoli, and cauliflower

Snack: Cup of diced cantaloupe

Day 4

Breakfast: Savory oats seasoned with cinnamon, a touch of ground coriander, ground cloves, ground ginger, a sprinkle of nutmeg and ground cardamom. Drizzle with a little real maple syrup which has a molecule with anti-inflammatory properties.

Lunch: Roasted sweet potato cut into strips like fries and served with avocado dip for a surprisingly delicious pairing

Dinner: Roasted garlic salmon with steamed cauliflower

Snack: Bell pepper strips with guacamole

Day 5

Breakfast: Pineapple smoothie made with green tea, kale, pineapple, frozen mango chunks, a tsp. of fresh ginger, and a pinch of turmeric

Lunch: Roasted red pepper and sweet potato soup

Dinner: Baked cod with pecan rosemary topping, and steamed green beans,

Snack: Cup of cherries

Day 6

Breakfast: Spinach and mushroom frittata

Lunch: Fruit salad made from your favorite in-season fruits

Dinner: Bell peppers, mushrooms, onions and diced tomatoes with chicken breast chunks, season with cayenne pepper for a little zip. Serve with quinoa

Snack: Dark chocolate

Day 7

Breakfast: Oatmeal seasoned with turmeric topped with plenty of colorful berries. Unique but delicious.

Lunch: Miso soup with gluten-free noodles

Dinner: Turkey and quinoa stuffed bell peppers

Snack: A serving of almonds

Conclusion

Thanks for making reading *Anti-Inflammatory Diet: Make these simple, inexpensive changes to your diet and start feeling better within 24 hours!*, let's hope it was informative and able to provide you with all of the tools you need to achieve your goals whatever they may be.

If the effects of chronic inflammation are robbing you of the joy of living because of pain, fatigue, weight gain or other health issues, it's time to take charge of your health. Now that you've read this book you are equipped to take steps toward healing. You've seen the statistics. Embrace the hope found in these pages and be proactive. Set a goal to consume less processed and fast foods and more fresh foods plentiful in fruits and vegetables. If you really want to see improvement, focus on health and healing, and that means thinking about every bite of food you take to get to your goal.

Don't be afraid to give up those favorite processed foods. They might taste good, but think about what you're really eating. Things like inflammation-triggering preservatives, artificial flavorings, and colorings, and then ask yourself if you want to still eat them. Don't think of it as depriving yourself, but instead think of it as empowering yourself to live healthier and pain-free. You don't have to be a slave to foods that aren't good for you, and you don't have to be controlled by pain or poor health.

Enjoy a piece of chocolate, and a cup of coffee and feel guilt free as you learn to eliminate inflammation triggering foods from your diet. You'll find a sense of freedom in just feeling better. Yes, it can take time, but remember it took time for the inflammation your fighting to become chronic. Each day is worth the fight toward better health, and now you have the arsenal at your fingertips to fight it.

Finally, if you found this book useful in any way, a review on Amazon is always appreciated!

Yours in health,
Jason Michaels

CPSIA information can be obtained
at www.ICGtesting.com
Printed in the USA
BVHW042348091221
623633BV00010B/551